Contents

A Comprehensive Guide for Understanding Dementia 2

What Is Dementia? 3

Why it is an important topic to discuss: 5

Brief Overview of What This Book Will Cover: 6

Understanding of Dementia: 8

Various Risk Factors for Developing Dementia: 10

Pathophysiology of Dementia: 12

Different Stages of Dementia Progression: 14

Symptoms of Dementia: 15

Behavioral Symptoms: 18

Diagnosis and Assessment for Dementia: 22

21 Techniques To Stop Dementia: 26

Conclusion 34

Stay Positive From Dementia And Alzheimer's Journal....35

A Comprehensive Guide for Understanding Dementia

Dementia is a syndrome of irreversible impairment of memory, thinking, judgment, insight, or mood. The most common form of dementia is Alzheimer's disease (AD), which causes behavioral and cognitive changes that can be disruptive and lead to loss of personal care. It is distinguished by a deterioration in cognitive abilities that might interfere with everyday living and frequently affects memory, reasoning, language, and problem-solving ability. Dementia is a general term embracing many different disorders, and it is currently thought that it has two main forms: Alzheimer's disease and vascular dementia.

Dementia affects people differently, with various symptoms, consequences, and prognosis. Awareness of these differences will enhance the chances of identifying what the patient is experiencing and ensuring appropriate treatment is applied. Since dementia can vary significantly in presentation from person to person and even at different stages in an individual's life, obtaining an individualized assessment from a neuropsychologist or psychiatrist with experience with the disorder is advisable.

Dementia is a syndrome of irreversible impairment of memory, thinking, judgment, insight, or mood. The most common form of dementia is Alzheimer's disease (AD), which causes behavioral and cognitive changes that can be disruptive and lead to loss of personal care. In this comprehensive guide, we will delve into the multifaceted aspects of dementia, seeking to provide a deep understanding of what dementia is, why it is crucial to discuss it, and the range of topics this book will cover.

What Is Dementia?

Disorders of thinking, memory, language and behavior caused by brain damage. Memory loss and difficulties in reasoning are the most frequent symptoms. An acute or chronic condition is often progressive, either primary or secondary. Alzheimer's disease is the most common cause of dementia among older adults. Vascular dementia develops due to a series of strokes in the brain. Each case presents different symptoms depending on the location and extent of brain damage, age, s*x, environment and genetic predisposition.

Dementia can significantly influence a person's capacity to live an independent and fulfilled life. It is a progressive disease, and, for many people, it can mark the end of their psychosocial career. The resources available to help each person with Alzheimer's disease or dementia require a commitment from all members of society, especially those who live with them. Every individual may need special care and assistance in dealing with their needs to preserve their dignity and independence.

The main challenges are to prevent the complications that may arise, such as infections and burns, and to enable them to stay in the familiar environment of their homes for as long as possible. For those who cannot care for themselves, a team of trained carers must be available to help them with their daily lives. In this book, we will try to shed light on the different aspects that social workers and others concerned may have about dementia.

Why it is an important topic to discuss:

Dementia discussion is necessary for numerous reasons. The vast majority of people affected by dementia live in their own homes. This requires a change in the way the family interacts with one another. When one family member develops dementia, it can be a struggle to keep up with this person's needs (especially in an isolated home), and it is necessary to create awareness within the family about how to support this person's cognitive abilities best.

Another important aspect of dementia discussion is education. To learn more about dementia or be aware of this condition, many people will want to learn more about what it is like for sufferers and their families. This can help people not affected by dementia feel more comfortable speaking with someone who has experienced it.

In addition, this information can be useful for doctors, nurses, and other healthcare professionals who may need a better understanding of the condition to assist affected people better. In some cases, this can even help people with dementia live independently for longer periods. The ability to discuss the condition may also help people with dementia maintain their boundaries.

Brief Overview of What This Book Will Cover:

This book is organized to give an in-depth examination of dementia from several perspectives:

1. Dementia Understanding: In this part, we will look at the many aspects of dementia, beginning with an overview of its numerous types, such as Alzheimer's disease, vascular dementia, Lewy body dementia, and others. We will also review the risk factors for acquiring dementia, the biology of the disease, and the many phases of dementia progression.

2. Symptoms of Dementia: We will delve into the common symptoms of dementia, such as memory loss and behavioral changes. We will also discuss the signs and symptoms of dementia unique to different types of dementia, including vascular dementia, Lewy body dementia, and others.

3. Social Impact: This part will look at how those with family members with Alzheimer's disease or other types of dementia experience this condition, including making changes to daily activities that are necessary or beneficial for their loved ones.

4. Dementia Treatment: This section will examine several considerations for possible treatments for people with dementia. We will look at the role of psychosocial therapy and other therapies, such as physical rehabilitation and medication. We will also cover how the symptoms of dementia may need to be managed to improve a person's quality of life.

5. Dementia Care: In this section, we will look at how those who care for a loved one with dementia work with their family members and professionals to provide care for them. We will examine how individuals with dementia can benefit from this type of assistance and what activities may benefit them.

6. Diagnosis and Assessment for Dementia: This section will cover the diagnostic testing needs for people with suspected dementia. We will examine how an Alzheimer's diagnosis is made and how other types of dementia can be diagnosed. We will also examine the possible treatments for different types of dementia and what kinds of support a person may need to manage their condition.

7. Dementia Prevention: In this part, we will look at lifestyle changes that can benefit those at risk of dementia. We will also consider a few strategies that can limit inflammation and cellular damage in the brain, as well as strategies that can be put in place to help people maintain their mental ability throughout their lives.

Understanding of Dementia:

Overview of Various Forms of Dementia:

Dementia is not a disorder that fits everybody. There are several types, each with its own set of qualities and reasons. The following are some of the most frequent types of dementia:

1. Alzheimer's disease:

The most common kind of dementia, Alzheimer's disease, accounts for the vast majority of cases. There is an abnormal buildup of a protein known as amyloid-β plaques in the brain, which destroy nerve cells responsible for learning and memory. Over time, this causes memory loss, confusion, and eventually death. Alzheimer's disease is often confused with senility, which can be caused by other factors such as medication for blood pressure or other illnesses.

2. Vascular dementia:

In contrast to Alzheimer's disease, vascular dementia occurs when blood flow to the brain is interrupted or reduced due to a problem with the arteries or blood vessels in the brain. This can lead to symptoms like memory loss and confusion. It can be caused by damage, including strokes and high blood pressure. It appears variable depending on the brain regions damaged and can cause issues with thinking, problem-solving, and other cognitive tasks.

3. Dementia with Lewy bodies:

Unlike most other forms of dementia, Lewy body dementia is characterized by clumps of a protein called alpha-synuclein that are found throughout the brain. This protein builds up as plaques or clusters, which causes nerve damage that leads to memory loss and confusion. Because this protein also affects neurons that respond to visual information, people with this form of dementia may develop visual hallucinations or other symptoms related to vision problems. This form of dementia also has an increased risk for falls and other movement-related issues.

4. Frontotemporal Dementia:

Problems with language, memory, planning, and problem-solving characterize frontotemporal dementia. It is caused by damage to the frontal areas of the brain. This includes areas of the brain that control speech and language and areas that govern how we understand emotional expression and social behavior. Because these are so important to daily functioning, it is often difficult to identify this form of dementia in people under age 60.

Various Risk Factors for Developing Dementia:

Understanding the risk factors for dementia is essential for prevention and early detection. While age is still the major risk factor for dementia, there are various other factors to consider:

1. Age: The greatest significant risk factor for acquiring dementia is age. The risk of dementia rises with age, especially beyond 65.

2. Gender: Women are at a higher risk for dementia than men, even after accounting for the effects of aging. Women tend to develop Alzheimer's disease about 20 years earlier than men. In addition, women tend to have a greater chance of developing Lewy body dementia and vascular dementia, although they are less likely to have Alzheimer's disease.

3. Genetics: Some studies have shown that a high genetic risk for dementia can also make a person susceptible to an early onset of dementia. This tends to be much less common, but it is still possible.

4. Diet: Several studies have looked at the link between specific types of food and dementia risk.

5. Cardiovascular Health: Several studies have found that people with a history of cardiovascular problems are more likely to develop issues like vascular dementia. This includes those with heart attacks, strokes, and other conditions.

6. Environmental toxins: It is important to help reduce exposure to environmental toxins such as lead paint, which could cause brain damage or dementia symptoms. In addition, avoiding smoking can help prevent vascular dementia and improve cardiovascular health.

7. Lack of exercise: Studies have shown that people who do not engage in moderate physical activity are more likely to develop age-related cognitive decline and be more likely to develop Alzheimer's disease later on in life.

Pathophysiology of Dementia:

Dementia causes differ based on the kind of dementia. However, several similar characteristics underpin most cases of cognitive decline:

1. Damage to Brain Cells: In most kinds of dementia, brain cells (neurons) and connections (synapses) are significantly lost. This cell injury interrupts normal brain function and inhibits cognitive functions.

2. Loss of Synapses: In the affected areas of the brain, there is a loss of synapses, a type of connection. This leads to a reduction in the ability to process information.

3. Abnormal Chemical Switches: In Alzheimer's disease, different chemicals are misregulated in the brain related to cognitive function, leading to memory loss and other symptoms. The exact reasons for this have yet to be fully understood. Still, it is thought that it occurs because these chemicals normally help control communication between neurons and other brain parts. These may be disrupted by inflammation or other factors that cause lasting damage in people with Alzheimer's disease.

4. Blood Flow Impairments: An additional problem in Alzheimer's disease is the depletion of oxygen and nutrients to the brain, causing the neurons to die. This refers to what's called hypoperfusion rather than hypoxia. Blood flow problems can also occur in vascular dementia due to problems with blood vessels in the brain.

5. Neuroinflammation: Inflammation is a normal body response when it has been injured or is attacked by pathogens and other factors. However, when this reaction occurs within the brain or spinal cord, it can cause damage or even death of neurons.

Different Stages of Dementia Progression:

Dementia normally proceeds in phases, with the pace of advancement varying from person to person. The phases are frequently defined as follows:

1. MCI (Mild Cognitive Impairment): People with MCI can still function normally. However, they may show a decreased attention span, a poor ability to reason and solve problems, and other signs of subtle memory impairment.

2. Early Stage: This describes the middle stage of dementia, where people may show more pronounced memory and reasoning problems and behavioral issues like agitation or aggression.

3. Late Stage: People will have significant problems with memory and the ability to think clearly. It also usually includes some behaviour symptoms like aggression.

4. Middle Stage: People at this stage of dementia typically have much more severe symptoms than those in the late stage. However, they still show some ability to perform daily tasks, such as bathing and dressing.

5. End-Stage: At the end-stage of dementia, not only are people unable to perform basic tasks like bathing and dressing, but they also cannot think enough to reason with others and may have significant mood swings or other behavioral issues.

Understanding the many types of dementia, recognizing risk factors, comprehending the pathophysiological processes involved, and being aware of the phases of development are critical for caregivers, healthcare professionals, and dementia patients.

Symptoms of Dementia:

Dementia is a symptom affecting an individual's cognitive, behavioral, and psychological functioning.

These symptoms frequently worsen with time and vary in intensity based on the kind of dementia and the individual's features. Understanding these signs is critical for diagnosing and treating people who are impacted.

Cognitive Symptoms:

Dementia is characterized by cognitive symptoms, often including deficits in thinking, memory, and other intellectual capacities. Among the most prevalent cognitive symptoms are:

1. Loss of Memory: One of the most common symptoms among people with dementia is a significant loss of memory, which often includes a decreased ability to remember recent events and faces. However, some people with dementia have problems recalling even older events from their past.

2. Impaired Judgement: The other most common cognitive symptom of dementia is faulty judgment. This can manifest itself in various ways, including poor creativity and judgment in decision-making, problems with understanding concepts such as time and money, and poor spatial skills.

3. Difficulty Learning New Things: Another common cognitive symptom of dementia is a hard time learning new things, such as information related to everyday living skills or new hobbies. This may include learning new languages or a new instrument, but it could also be more severe if the full scope of knowledge has been lost.

4. Confusion occurs when a person with dementia experiences problems with memory or problem-solving and comprehension, leading to difficulties understanding relevant information.

5. Inability to focus: This is often confused with confusion, but it is a different condition that comes from difficulty finding mental stimulation. This can include an inability to plan or organize new activities and a lack of interest in engaging in new and interesting activities.

6. Disorientation: This is often considered an extreme form of confusion because disoriented people cannot respond or answer questions about their surroundings or the time of day. They may also be unable to recognize people around them and have problems recognizing themselves.

Behavioral Symptoms:

Dementia is considered a chronic rather than an acute condition because it develops over time. Rather than causing sudden changes in behavior or personality, it is often characterized by behavior problems that gradually develop over longer periods. Therefore, behavioral symptoms are common following the onset of dementia. They include the following:

1. Agitation and Aggression: Agitation is a common behavioral symptom that occurs in many people with dementia when they can't express themselves verbally. This may include screaming, yelling, crying, or even physical violence like kicking or throwing objects. Agitation can also be expressed as pacing or walking around for long periods without stopping.

2. Restlessness: This is an all-encompassing symptom that describes uncontrolled and persistently increasing restlessness or stress, which can be expressed in numerous ways. This may include fidgeting, pacing for extended periods, excessive rocking activities, or unnecessary movement throughout the day.

3. Difficulty Sleeping: Difficulty sleeping is another common behavioral symptom of dementia because people with dementia have trouble falling or staying asleep at night. This may include vivid dreams and sleepwalking.

4. Difficulty with Pain: The inability to control pain can cause people with dementia to continue doing things they know are harmful to their overall health or safety daily despite clear signs of pain from others.

5. Personality Changes: People with dementia may experience significant personality changes over time as they develop behavioral symptoms. These may include becoming surly, hostile, or paranoid, even when they don't have any reason to be. However, these personality changes can also include personality regression that removes new behaviors or traits that developed in the previous stages of dementia.

Psychological Symptoms:

The following psychological symptoms are commonly considered the least severe symptoms of dementia because they aren't typically as detrimental to the individual's quality of life. However, they can also lead to depression and social isolation if left untreated:

1. Problems with Communication: People with dementia may have problems communicating verbally or nonverbally, which is often a symptom of language and motor skills impairment. This can include speaking slowly or slurred word choice, an inability to respond verbally when asked a question, or a struggle to understand questions or instructions from others.

2. Emotional Instability: People with dementia may experience mood changes that are difficult to describe but noticeable by others who know them well. These changes can manifest as extreme irritability, a lack of emotional control, or even a loss of inhibitions due to difficulty understanding social norms. This may include acting out in socially inappropriate ways like yelling, inappropriate sexual advances, or speaking inappropriately in public.

3. Delusions: This is uncommon when people with dementia are confronted with reality and persistently believe something untrue. Delusions may include beliefs of persecution, witchcraft, immortality, fortune-telling skills, or other things that are not true.

4. Depression: People with dementia may develop depression when other symptoms of the condition become difficult to cope with daily. This can include feelings of worthlessness, guilt, or persistent sadness that limit their ability to enjoy activities and relationships that were once important to them. Depression among people with dementia is often treated with antidepressants or other mood-altering drugs.

5. Hallucinations: This refers to a condition where people who are impaired by some aspect of their dementia believe they are experiencing sights, sounds, textures, emotions, or tastes that aren't present in their environment. Hallucinations may include seeing people who aren't there, or hearing sounds most people cannot hear.

6. Paranoia: People with dementia may misinterpret situations in the environment and develop paranoid delusions, including beliefs that others are out to harm, embarrass, or humiliate them. Even when this is not the case, they may become convinced that others are giving them undeserved harsh treatment or disrespect.

7. Personality Changes: One of the most difficult symptoms for family members and caregivers of people with dementia is the change in personality over time. These changes are often subtle and slow to develop but can become noticeable over time. These changes can include a loss of inhibitions or the tendency to act in uncharacteristic ways of the person before their dementia took hold.

Diagnosis and Assessment for Dementia:

Diagnosis of dementia is a difficult procedure that involves a detailed assessment of a person's cognitive and functional skills. Healthcare experts use various tests and examinations to establish the presence of dementia and uncover its underlying etiology. We will look at the most important aspects of diagnosing and assessing dementia.

1. **Clinical assessments:** To obtain information concerning cognitive changes, behavior, and symptoms, a healthcare professional conducts a full clinical evaluation that includes a medical history, physical examination, and interviews with the individual and their family.

2. **Mental status examination:** This test involves observing the cognitive and motor skills of the person being evaluated to determine how well their mental processes work. This can be performed using assessment tools and skills to provide an overview of the person's mental health.

3. **Laboratory tests:** Generally, these tests are not required for diagnosing dementia but may be useful if there is suspicion that an underlying medical condition could be a contributing factor to the development of dementia symptoms.

4. Magnetic Resonance Imaging (MRI): An MRI scan provides detailed pictures of the brain's anatomy and can be used to detect the presence of certain lesions or tumors that could be related to dementia. However, most people with dementia don't experience changes in their brain tissue, so this test may not provide useful information in most cases.

5. Neuropsychological Testing: A Neuropsychological test is a standardized clinical tool that can help evaluate the cognitive skills of an individual affected by dementia. This includes tests to determine general cognitive functioning and memory, language, attention, perception, and other functions. These tools can be useful in determining how quickly dementia progresses or whether there is evidence of frontal lobe damage or Alzheimer's disease present in cases where other medical conditions are suspected as the cause of dementia.

6. Cognitive function: The most basic indicator that a person has Alzheimer's Disease is brain atrophy or shrinkage caused by damage to the tissues surrounding brain cells. People with dementia also become less able to perform basic everyday tasks like dressing or bathing themselves, often requiring help from family members. A Health Professional can use the generic version of the Standardized Mini-Mental State Examination, a standardized clinical tool to assess the cognitive skills of individuals affected by dementia.

7. Genetic Testing: No definitive test is available to determine the presence of dementia due to Alzheimer's Disease, but a genetic testing procedure can confirm if the person has the genetic markers indicating an increased risk for developing Alzheimer's Disease later in life. However, most cases of dementia are not caused by Alzheimer's Disease, and a positive diagnosis could result in undue anxiety or distress in the affected individual.

8. Psychiatric Evaluation: Often, families are concerned about the possibility of a mental illness being the underlying cause of their loved one's dementia. A psychiatric evaluation can help to rule out the presence of such an illness by examining the person for symptoms that might suggest an underlying mental health problem. By providing a professional diagnosis, people with dementia and their caregivers can have more realistic expectations about what is happening to them and how they should be treated.

9. Occupational Therapy: Occupational therapy can help improve daily living skills for people with dementia. This type of therapy focuses on teaching new skills that improve the person's physical mobility and increase their independence. The goal is to help people maintain their quality of life after they develop dementia.

10. Physical Therapy: Physical therapy is another therapeutic option that can be helpful for people with Alzheimer's and other types of dementia. Occupational therapists often work with patients who are beginning to lose the ability to perform certain basic daily tasks like feeding themselves, washing themselves, dressing, or manipulating everyday objects.

21 Techniques To Stop Dementia:

While there is no treatment for dementia, research has shown measures that may help minimize the chance of acquiring dementia or halt its course. These methods are aimed at preserving brain health and overall well-being:

1. Physical Exercise: For people with dementia, physical exercise can help to combat possible problems related to weight gain and circulation issues. It has also been shown in studies to improve memory, learning, and mental function and reduce depression symptoms. The ideal type of physical activity for individuals affected by dementia is aerobic exercise.

2. Mental Stimulation: According to experts, this is one of the most effective ways to slow down cognitive decline in individuals with dementia. This can include playing board games, doing crossword puzzles, reading newspapers and books or watching movies.

3. Healthy Diet: A diet with a regular supply of essential vitamins and minerals can help slow cognitive function deterioration among people with dementia. According to research, a Mediterranean-style diet rich in fruits and vegetables has produced positive results regarding mental sharpness and brain health.

4. Social interaction: People with dementia may have trouble communicating their thoughts and feelings but still need socialization. Family members and friends can help minimize the risk of depression and anxiety by engaging them in activities that stimulate them cognitively and emotionally.

5. Mental Stimulants: These may be used to slow down the progression of Alzheimer's Disease or at least alleviate some of its symptoms.

6. Pain Relief: Dementia is one of the most painful syndromes that affect the elderly. Painful symptoms are experienced in many body parts, including the lower back and joints. A combination of drugs and exercise can help relieve pain and improve mobility for people with dementia, as well as decrease muscle tenderness, which is a common side effect of pain medications.

7. Exercise For The Lumbar Spine: Using a walker or wheelchair may be more effective than using physical restraints in managing a person's basic activities of daily living, but they do not allow for regular exercise that helps strengthen muscles around the spine. Physical therapists can design a program that uses resistance and balance exercises to strengthen the lower back. These exercises will also prevent muscle spasms and maintain overall spinal health.

8. Managing Sleep Problems: People with dementia may have trouble sleeping due to frequent waking, agitation or anxiety. Healthcare professionals can recommend herbal remedies and hormone supplements to improve sleep quality for people with dementia.

9. Massage Therapy: This is another form of physical therapy that helps improve circulation and reduce muscle tension and pain in people with dementia. Massage increases blood flow to the brain, improves brain function, relieves mental stress, reduces anxiety and depression symptoms, and improves overall mood in patients with dementia.

10. Weight Management: Weight gain is one of the most common side effects of Alzheimer's Disease. Other common side effects of dementia include dehydration, dry skin and hair loss. In addition to regular physical exercise, a healthy diet that starts with a breakfast rich in protein and cholesterol and ends with a dinner rich in carbohydrates is best for maintaining healthy blood pressure.

11. Pain Medications: Aside from the symptoms associated with pain, such as restless sleep, excessive sweating and muscle spasms, people with dementia may also experience other symptoms, such as anxiety or depression due to these symptoms. Pain relievers may help reduce this stress on the person suffering from these problems and help them maintain their overall health.

12. Stay Hydrated: For people with dementia, dehydration can make them more forgetful and confused, so it is important to encourage them to drink at least eight glasses of water daily. Water is necessary for general health, including brain function.

13. Stay socially active: Like many other mental conditions, the best treatment for dementia involves encouraging the affected person to participate in activities that stimulate the brain and improve their quality of life.

14. Keep the mind sharp: According to research, keeping the mind active through reading or doing crossword puzzles helps to keep it sharp as well as slowing down mental deterioration in people with Alzheimer's Disease. It also helps to prevent or delay memory loss due to age-related brain deterioration.

15. Omega-3 Fatty Acids: These may help to reduce the risk of cognitive decline and memory loss among people with Alzheimer's Disease. Omega-3 fatty acids are essential because humans can't produce them independently; they must be obtained from foods or supplements.

16. Language Training: This is another effective way to keep the mind sharp and slow mental deterioration. People with dementia often have difficulty processing verbal and written information due to diminished brain function. Still, if their language skills improve, they can better communicate with friends and family. Regular practice will also prevent depression or anxiety that is brought about by an inability to communicate effectively and socialize with others.

17. Antioxidant-Rich Foods: These are high in antioxidants that may help slow down the progression of Alzheimer's Disease by preventing damage to cells that contain lipofuscin. This damage may eventually cause the formation of plaques and tangles in the brain.

18. Vitamin D: This vitamin is good for bone and brain health but may also prevent premature death due to dementia among people who have not previously suffered from this condition.

19. Engage in Lifelong Learning: This is another effective way to keep the mind sharp and slow mental deterioration. People with dementia often have difficulty processing verbal and written information due to diminished brain function. Still, if their language skills improve, they can better communicate with friends and family. Regular practice will also prevent depression or anxiety that is brought about by an inability to communicate effectively and socialize with others.

20. Stay socially active: Like many other mental conditions, the best treatment for dementia involves encouraging the affected person to participate in activities that stimulate the brain and improve their quality of life.

21. Keep the mind sharp: According to research, keeping the mind active through reading or doing crossword puzzles helps to keep it sharp as well as slowing down mental deterioration in people with Alzheimer's Disease. It also helps to prevent or delay memory loss due to age-related brain deterioration.

Conclusion

To summarize, dementia is a difficult and diverse disorder affecting millions globally. It is an important public health problem since it involves a wide spectrum of cognitive, behavioral, and psychiatric symptoms. This book has looked at several elements of dementia, including its types, risk factors, pathogenesis, and phases of development. Understanding the many types of dementia, from Alzheimer's to vascular dementia, is critical for proper diagnosis and personalized therapy. Recognizing dementia risk factors, such as age, genetics, and lifestyle choices, is critical for prevention and early intervention. With the help of these tips, you can manage the effects of Alzheimer's Disease and improve your quality of life.

Important Note

Please consult with the relevant doctor or expert first before doing or taking any steps or action do not rely on our or in this case any book.

Stay Positivity Journal

DATE: _____

Today I'm grateful because :
- _____
- _____
- _____

Today's Positive Affirmations / Quotes
- _____
- _____
- _____
- _____

Water Tracker
☐ 1L ☐ 2L ☐ 3L

Today I'm feeling ◯ ← **Emoji**

Notes / reminders:

Something I'm proud of
- _____
- _____
- _____
- _____

Tomorrow I look forward to
- _____
- _____
- _____
- _____

Stay Positivity Journal

DATE: _____

Today I'm grateful because :
- _____
- _____
- _____

Today's Positive Affirmations / Quotes
- _____
- _____
- _____
- _____

Water Tracker
☐ 1L   ☐ 2L   ☐ 3L

Today I'm feeling ◯ **Emoji**

Notes / reminders:

Something I'm proud of
- _____
- _____
- _____
- _____

Tomorrow I look forward to
- _____
- _____
- _____
- _____

Stay Positivity Journal

DATE: _____

Today I'm grateful because :
- _____
- _____
- _____

Today's Positive Affirmations / Quotes
- _____
- _____
- _____
- _____

Water Tracker
- ☐ 1L ☐ 2L ☐ 3L

Today I'm feeling ◯ → **Emoji**

Notes / reminders:

Something I'm proud of
- _____
- _____
- _____
- _____

Tomorrow I look forward to
- _____
- _____
- _____
- _____

Stay Positivity Journal

DATE: _____

Today I'm grateful because :
- _____
- _____
- _____

Today's Positive Affirmations / Quotes
- _____
- _____
- _____
- _____

Water Tracker

☐ 1L ☐ 2L ☐ 3L

Today I'm feeling ⭕ **Emoji**

Notes / reminders:

Something I'm proud of
- _____
- _____
- _____
- _____

Tomorrow I look forward to
- _____
- _____
- _____
- _____

Stay Positivity Journal

DATE: _____

Today I'm grateful because :
- _____
- _____
- _____

Today's Positive Affirmations / Quotes
- _____
- _____
- _____
- _____

Water Tracker
- ☐ 1L ☐ 2L ☐ 3L

Today I'm feeling ◯ Emoji

Notes / reminders:

Something I'm proud of
- _____
- _____
- _____
- _____

Tomorrow I look forward to
- _____
- _____
- _____
- _____

Stay Positivity Journal

DATE: _____

Today I'm grateful because :
- _____
- _____
- _____

Today's Positive Affirmations / Quotes
- _____
- _____
- _____
- _____

Water Tracker
- ☐ 1L   ☐ 2L   ☐ 3L

Today I'm feeling ◯ ← **Emoji**

Notes / reminders:

Something I'm proud of
- _____
- _____
- _____
- _____

Tomorrow I look forward to
- _____
- _____
- _____
- _____

Stay Positivity Journal

DATE: _____

Today I'm grateful because :

- _____
- _____
- _____

Today's Positive Affirmations / Quotes

- _____
- _____
- _____
- _____

Water Tracker

☐ 1L   ☐ 2L   ☐ 3L

Today I'm feeling ◯ **Emoji**

Notes / reminders:

Something I'm proud of

- _____
- _____
- _____
- _____

Tomorrow I look forward to

- _____
- _____
- _____
- _____

Stay Positivity Journal

DATE: _____

Today I'm grateful because :
- _____
- _____
- _____

Today's Positive Affirmations / Quotes
- _____
- _____
- _____
- _____

Water Tracker
- ☐ 1L ☐ 2L ☐ 3L

Today I'm feeling ◯ → **Emoji**

Notes / reminders:

Something I'm proud of
- _____
- _____
- _____
- _____

Tomorrow I look forward to
- _____
- _____
- _____
- _____

Stay Positivity Journal

DATE: _____

Today I'm grateful because :
- _____
- _____
- _____

Today's Positive Affirmations / Quotes
- _____
- _____
- _____
- _____

Water Tracker

☐ 1L ☐ 2L ☐ 3L

Today I'm feeling ◯ **Emoji**

Notes / reminders:

Something I'm proud of
- _____
- _____
- _____
- _____

Tomorrow I look forward to
- _____
- _____
- _____
- _____

Stay Positivity Journal

DATE: _____

Today I'm grateful because :
- _____
- _____
- _____

Today's Positive Affirmations / Quotes
- _____
- _____
- _____
- _____

Water Tracker
- ☐ 1L   ☐ 2L   ☐ 3L

Today I'm feeling ◯ ← Emoji

Notes / reminders:

Something I'm proud of
- _____
- _____
- _____
- _____

Tomorrow I look forward to
- _____
- _____
- _____
- _____

Stay Positivity Journal

DATE: _____

Today I'm grateful because :
- _____
- _____
- _____

Today's Positive Affirmations / Quotes
- _____
- _____
- _____
- _____

Water Tracker
- ☐ 1L ☐ 2L ☐ 3L

Today I'm feeling ◯ **Emoji**

Notes / reminders:

Something I'm proud of
- _____
- _____
- _____
- _____

Tomorrow I look forward to
- _____
- _____
- _____
- _____

Stay Positivity Journal

DATE: _____

Today I'm grateful because :
- _____
- _____
- _____

Today's Positive Affirmations / Quotes
- _____
- _____
- _____
- _____

Water Tracker
- ☐ 1L   ☐ 2L   ☐ 3L

Today I'm feeling ⭕ ← Emoji

Notes / reminders:

Something I'm proud of
- _____
- _____
- _____
- _____

Tomorrow I look forward to
- _____
- _____
- _____
- _____

Stay Positivity Journal

DATE: _____

Today I'm grateful because :
- _____
- _____
- _____

Today's Positive Affirmations / Quotes
- _____
- _____
- _____
- _____

Water Tracker
- ☐ 1L ☐ 2L ☐ 3L

Today I'm feeling ◯ ← Emoji

Notes / reminders:

Something I'm proud of
- _____
- _____
- _____
- _____

Tomorrow I look forward to
- _____
- _____
- _____
- _____

Stay Positivity Journal

DATE: _____

Today I'm grateful because :
- _____
- _____
- _____

Today's Positive Affirmations / Quotes
- _____
- _____
- _____
- _____

Water Tracker
☐ 1L ☐ 2L ☐ 3L

Today I'm feeling ⃝ → Emoji

Notes / reminders:

Something I'm proud of
- _____
- _____
- _____
- _____

Tomorrow I look forward to
- _____
- _____
- _____
- _____

Stay Positivity Journal

DATE: _____

Today I'm grateful because :
- _____
- _____
- _____

Today's Positive Affirmations / Quotes
- _____
- _____
- _____
- _____

Water Tracker
☐ 1L   ☐ 2L   ☐ 3L

Today I'm feeling ◯ **Emoji**

Notes / reminders:

Something I'm proud of
- _____
- _____
- _____
- _____

Tomorrow I look forward to
- _____
- _____
- _____
- _____

Stay Positivity Journal

DATE: _____

Today I'm grateful because :

- _____
- _____
- _____

Today's Positive Affirmations / Quotes

- _____
- _____
- _____
- _____

Water Tracker

☐ 1L   ☐ 2L   ☐ 3L

Today I'm feeling ◯ **Emoji**

Notes / reminders:

Something I'm proud of

- _____
- _____
- _____
- _____

Tomorrow I look forward to

- _____
- _____
- _____
- _____

Stay Positivity Journal

DATE: _____

Today I'm grateful because :
- _____
- _____
- _____

Today's Positive Affirmations / Quotes
- _____
- _____
- _____
- _____

Water Tracker
- ☐ 1L ☐ 2L ☐ 3L

Today I'm feeling ⟲ Emoji

Notes / reminders:

Something I'm proud of
- _____
- _____
- _____
- _____

Tomorrow I look forward to
- _____
- _____
- _____
- _____

Stay Positivity Journal

DATE: _____

Today I'm grateful because :
- _____
- _____
- _____

Today's Positive Affirmations / Quotes
- _____
- _____
- _____
- _____

Water Tracker
☐ 1L ☐ 2L ☐ 3L

Today I'm feeling ◯ → **Emoji**

Notes / reminders:

Something I'm proud of
- _____
- _____
- _____
- _____

Tomorrow I look forward to
- _____
- _____
- _____
- _____

Stay Positivity Journal

DATE: _____

Today I'm grateful because :
- _____
- _____
- _____

Today's Positive Affirmations / Quotes
- _____
- _____
- _____
- _____

Water Tracker
☐ 1L ☐ 2L ☐ 3L

Today I'm feeling ⭕ → **Emoji**

Notes / reminders:

Something I'm proud of
- _____
- _____
- _____
- _____

Tomorrow I look forward to
- _____
- _____
- _____
- _____

Stay Positivity Journal

DATE: _____

Today I'm grateful because :
- _____
- _____
- _____

Today's Positive Affirmations / Quotes
- _____
- _____
- _____
- _____

Water Tracker
- ☐ 1L   ☐ 2L   ☐ 3L

Today I'm feeling ⟶ Emoji

Notes / reminders:

Something I'm proud of
- _____
- _____
- _____
- _____

Tomorrow I look forward to
- _____
- _____
- _____
- _____

Stay Positivity Journal

DATE: _____

Today I'm grateful because :
- _____
- _____
- _____

Today's Positive Affirmations / Quotes
- _____
- _____
- _____
- _____

Water Tracker
☐ 1L ☐ 2L ☐ 3L

Today I'm feeling ⭕ Emoji

Notes / reminders:

Something I'm proud of
- _____
- _____
- _____
- _____

Tomorrow I look forward to
- _____
- _____
- _____
- _____

Stay Positivity Journal

DATE: _____

Today I'm grateful because :
- _____
- _____
- _____

Today's Positive Affirmations / Quotes
- _____
- _____
- _____
- _____

Water Tracker
☐ 1L   ☐ 2L   ☐ 3L

Today I'm feeling ◯ → **Emoji**

Notes / reminders:

Something I'm proud of
- _____
- _____
- _____
- _____

Tomorrow I look forward to
- _____
- _____
- _____
- _____

Stay Positivity Journal

DATE: _____

Today I'm grateful because :

- _____
- _____
- _____

Today's Positive Affirmations / Quotes

- _____
- _____
- _____
- _____

Water Tracker

☐ 1L   ☐ 2L   ☐ 3L

Today I'm feeling → **Emoji**

Notes / reminders:

Something I'm proud of

- _____
- _____
- _____
- _____

Tomorrow I look forward to

- _____
- _____
- _____
- _____

Stay Positivity Journal

DATE: _____

Today I'm grateful because :
- _____
- _____
- _____

Today's Positive Affirmations / Quotes
- _____
- _____
- _____
- _____

Water Tracker
- ☐ 1L ☐ 2L ☐ 3L

Today I'm feeling ◯ → **Emoji**

Notes / reminders:

Something I'm proud of
- _____
- _____
- _____
- _____

Tomorrow I look forward to
- _____
- _____
- _____
- _____

Stay Positivity Journal

DATE: _____

Today I'm grateful because :
- _____
- _____
- _____

Today's Positive Affirmations / Quotes
- _____
- _____
- _____
- _____

Water Tracker
- ☐ 1L   ☐ 2L   ☐ 3L

Today I'm feeling ⟶ Emoji

Notes / reminders:

Something I'm proud of
- _____
- _____
- _____
- _____

Tomorrow I look forward to
- _____
- _____
- _____
- _____

Stay Positivity Journal

DATE: _____

Today I'm grateful because :
- _____
- _____
- _____

Today's Positive Affirmations / Quotes
- _____
- _____
- _____
- _____

Water Tracker
☐ 1L   ☐ 2L   ☐ 3L

Today I'm feeling ◯ ← Emoji

Notes / reminders:

Something I'm proud of
- _____
- _____
- _____
- _____

Tomorrow I look forward to
- _____
- _____
- _____
- _____

Stay Positivity Journal

DATE: _____

Today I'm grateful because :
- _____
- _____
- _____

Today's Positive Affirmations / Quotes
- _____
- _____
- _____
- _____

Water Tracker
☐ 1L ☐ 2L ☐ 3L

Today I'm feeling ◯ **Emoji**

Notes / reminders:

Something I'm proud of
- _____
- _____
- _____
- _____

Tomorrow I look forward to
- _____
- _____
- _____
- _____

Stay Positivity Journal

DATE: _____

Today I'm grateful because :
- _____
- _____
- _____

Today's Positive Affirmations / Quotes
- _____
- _____
- _____
- _____

Water Tracker
- ☐ 1L ☐ 2L ☐ 3L

Today I'm feeling ◯ ← Emoji

Notes / reminders:

Something I'm proud of
- _____
- _____
- _____
- _____

Tomorrow I look forward to
- _____
- _____
- _____
- _____

Stay Positivity Journal

DATE: _____

Today I'm grateful because :
- _____
- _____
- _____

Today's Positive Affirmations / Quotes
- _____
- _____
- _____
- _____

Water Tracker
☐ 1L   ☐ 2L   ☐ 3L

Today I'm feeling ◯ → **Emoji**

Notes / reminders:

Something I'm proud of
- _____
- _____
- _____
- _____

Tomorrow I look forward to
- _____
- _____
- _____
- _____

Stay Positivity Journal

DATE: _____

Today I'm grateful because :
- _____
- _____
- _____

Today's Positive Affirmations / Quotes
- _____
- _____
- _____
- _____

Water Tracker
- ☐ 1L ☐ 2L ☐ 3L

Today I'm feeling ◯ → Emoji

Notes / reminders:

Something I'm proud of
- _____
- _____
- _____
- _____

Tomorrow I look forward to
- _____
- _____
- _____
- _____

Stay Positivity Journal

DATE: _____

Today I'm grateful because :

- _____
- _____
- _____

Today's Positive Affirmations / Quotes

- _____
- _____
- _____
- _____

Water Tracker

☐ 1L   ☐ 2L   ☐ 3L

Today I'm feeling ◯ → Emoji

Notes / reminders:

Something I'm proud of

- _____
- _____
- _____

Tomorrow I look forward to

- _____
- _____
- _____
- _____

Stay Positivity Journal

DATE: _____

Today I'm grateful because :
- _____
- _____
- _____

Today's Positive Affirmations / Quotes
- _____
- _____
- _____
- _____

Water Tracker
- ☐ 1L   ☐ 2L   ☐ 3L

Today I'm feeling ◯ ← Emoji

Notes / reminders:

Something I'm proud of
- _____
- _____
- _____
- _____

Tomorrow I look forward to
- _____
- _____
- _____
- _____

Stay Positivity Journal

DATE: _____

Today I'm grateful because :

- _____
- _____
- _____

Today's Positive Affirmations / Quotes

- _____
- _____
- _____
- _____

Water Tracker

☐ 1L   ☐ 2L   ☐ 3L

Today I'm feeling ○ Emoji

Notes / reminders:

Something I'm proud of

- _____
- _____
- _____
- _____

Tomorrow I look forward to

- _____
- _____
- _____
- _____

Stay Positivity Journal

DATE: _____

Today I'm grateful because :
- _____
- _____
- _____

Today's Positive Affirmations / Quotes
- _____
- _____
- _____
- _____

Water Tracker
☐ 1L   ☐ 2L   ☐ 3L

Today I'm feeling ◯ **Emoji**

Notes / reminders:

Something I'm proud of
- _____
- _____
- _____
- _____

Tomorrow I look forward to
- _____
- _____
- _____
- _____

Stay Positivity Journal

DATE: _____

Today I'm grateful because :

- _____
- _____
- _____

Today's Positive Affirmations / Quotes

- _____
- _____
- _____
- _____

Water Tracker

☐ 1L   ☐ 2L   ☐ 3L

Today I'm feeling ⭕ → **Emoji**

Notes / reminders:

Something I'm proud of

- _____
- _____
- _____
- _____

Tomorrow I look forward to

- _____
- _____
- _____
- _____

Stay Positivity Journal

DATE: _____

Today I'm grateful because :
- _____
- _____
- _____

Today's Positive Affirmations / Quotes
- _____
- _____
- _____
- _____

Water Tracker
☐ 1L   ☐ 2L   ☐ 3L

Today I'm feeling ◯ ← **Emoji**

Notes / reminders:

Something I'm proud of
- _____
- _____
- _____
- _____

Tomorrow I look forward to
- _____
- _____
- _____
- _____

Stay Positivity Journal

DATE: _____

Today I'm grateful because :
- _____
- _____
- _____

Today's Positive Affirmations / Quotes
- _____
- _____
- _____
- _____

Water Tracker

☐ 1L   ☐ 2L   ☐ 3L

Today I'm feeling ◯ ← Emoji

Notes / reminders:

Something I'm proud of
- _____
- _____
- _____
- _____

Tomorrow I look forward to
- _____
- _____
- _____
- _____

Stay Positivity Journal

DATE: _____

Today I'm grateful because :
- _____
- _____
- _____

Today's Positive Affirmations / Quotes
- _____
- _____
- _____
- _____

Water Tracker

☐ 1L   ☐ 2L   ☐ 3L

Today I'm feeling ⭕ → **Emoji**

Notes / reminders:

Something I'm proud of
- _____
- _____
- _____
- _____

Tomorrow I look forward to
- _____
- _____
- _____
- _____

Stay Positivity Journal

DATE: _____

Today I'm grateful because :

- _____
- _____
- _____

Today's Positive Affirmations / Quotes

- _____
- _____
- _____
- _____

Water Tracker

☐ 1L   ☐ 2L   ☐ 3L

Today I'm feeling ◯ → **Emoji**

Notes / reminders:

Something I'm proud of

- _____
- _____
- _____
- _____

Tomorrow I look forward to

- _____
- _____
- _____
- _____

Stay Positivity Journal

DATE: _____

Today I'm grateful because :
- _____
- _____
- _____

Today's Positive Affirmations / Quotes
- _____
- _____
- _____
- _____

Water Tracker
☐ 1L   ☐ 2L   ☐ 3L

Today I'm feeling ◯ **Emoji**

Notes / reminders:

Something I'm proud of
- _____
- _____
- _____
- _____

Tomorrow I look forward to
- _____
- _____
- _____
- _____

Stay Positivity Journal

DATE: _____

Today I'm grateful because :
- _____
- _____
- _____

Today's Positive Affirmations / Quotes
- _____
- _____
- _____
- _____

Water Tracker
☐ 1L   ☐ 2L   ☐ 3L

Today I'm feeling ◯ ← Emoji

Notes / reminders:

Something I'm proud of
- _____
- _____
- _____
- _____

Tomorrow I look forward to
- _____
- _____
- _____
- _____

Stay Positivity Journal

DATE: _____

Today I'm grateful because :
- _____
- _____
- _____

Today's Positive Affirmations / Quotes
- _____
- _____
- _____
- _____

Water Tracker
- ☐ 1L   ☐ 2L   ☐ 3L

Today I'm feeling ◯ → Emoji

Notes / reminders:

Something I'm proud of
- _____
- _____
- _____
- _____

Tomorrow I look forward to
- _____
- _____
- _____
- _____

Stay Positivity Journal

DATE: _____

Today I'm grateful because :

- _____
- _____
- _____

Today's Positive Affirmations / Quotes

- _____
- _____
- _____
- _____

Water Tracker

☐ 1L ☐ 2L ☐ 3L

Today I'm feeling ◯ **Emoji**

Notes / reminders:

Something I'm proud of

- _____
- _____
- _____
- _____

Tomorrow I look forward to

- _____
- _____
- _____
- _____

Stay Positivity Journal

DATE: _____

Today I'm grateful because :
- _____
- _____
- _____

Today's Positive Affirmations / Quotes
- _____
- _____
- _____
- _____

Water Tracker

☐ 1L ☐ 2L ☐ 3L

Today I'm feeling ⟶ **Emoji**

Notes / reminders:

Something I'm proud of
- _____
- _____
- _____
- _____

Tomorrow I look forward to
- _____
- _____
- _____
- _____

Stay Positivity Journal

DATE: _____

Today I'm grateful because :
- _____
- _____
- _____

Today's Positive Affirmations / Quotes
- _____
- _____
- _____
- _____

Water Tracker
☐ 1L   ☐ 2L   ☐ 3L

Today I'm feeling ◯ Emoji

Notes / reminders:

Something I'm proud of
- _____
- _____
- _____
- _____

Tomorrow I look forward to
- _____
- _____
- _____
- _____

Stay Positivity Journal

DATE: _____

Today I'm grateful because :
- _____
- _____
- _____

Today's Positive Affirmations / Quotes
- _____
- _____
- _____
- _____

Water Tracker

☐ 1L ☐ 2L ☐ 3L

Today I'm feeling ⭕ **Emoji**

Notes / reminders:

Something I'm proud of
- _____
- _____
- _____
- _____

Tomorrow I look forward to
- _____
- _____
- _____
- _____

Stay Positivity Journal

DATE: _____

Today I'm grateful because :
- _____
- _____
- _____

Today's Positive Affirmations / Quotes
- _____
- _____
- _____
- _____

Water Tracker
- ☐ 1L ☐ 2L ☐ 3L

Today I'm feeling ◯ → Emoji

Notes / reminders:

Something I'm proud of
- _____
- _____
- _____
- _____

Tomorrow I look forward to
- _____
- _____
- _____
- _____

Stay Positivity Journal

DATE: _____

Today I'm grateful because :
- _____
- _____
- _____

Today's Positive Affirmations / Quotes
- _____
- _____
- _____
- _____

Water Tracker

☐ 1L   ☐ 2L   ☐ 3L

Today I'm feeling ◯ ↩ **Emoji**

Notes / reminders:

Something I'm proud of
- _____
- _____
- _____
- _____

Tomorrow I look forward to
- _____
- _____
- _____
- _____

Stay Positivity Journal

DATE: _____

Today I'm grateful because :
- _____
- _____
- _____

Today's Positive Affirmations / Quotes
- _____
- _____
- _____
- _____

Water Tracker
- ☐ 1L ☐ 2L ☐ 3L

Today I'm feeling ◯ ← Emoji

Notes / reminders:

Something I'm proud of
- _____
- _____
- _____
- _____

Tomorrow I look forward to
- _____
- _____
- _____
- _____

Stay Positivity Journal

DATE: _____

Today I'm grateful because :
- _____
- _____
- _____

Today's Positive Affirmations / Quotes
- _____
- _____
- _____
- _____

Water Tracker

☐ 1L   ☐ 2L   ☐ 3L

Today I'm feeling ◯ → Emoji

Notes / reminders:

Something I'm proud of
- _____
- _____
- _____
- _____

Tomorrow I look forward to
- _____
- _____
- _____
- _____

Stay Positivity Journal

DATE: _____

Today I'm grateful because :

- _____
- _____
- _____

Today's Positive Affirmations / Quotes

- _____
- _____
- _____
- _____

Water Tracker

☐ 1L ☐ 2L ☐ 3L

Today I'm feeling ⭕ → **Emoji**

Notes / reminders:

Something I'm proud of

- _____
- _____
- _____
- _____

Tomorrow I look forward to

- _____
- _____
- _____
- _____

Stay Positivity Journal

DATE: _____

Today I'm grateful because :
- _____
- _____
- _____

Today's Positive Affirmations / Quotes
- _____
- _____
- _____
- _____

Water Tracker
- ☐ 1L ☐ 2L ☐ 3L

Today I'm feeling ◯ → Emoji

Notes / reminders:

Something I'm proud of
- _____
- _____
- _____
- _____

Tomorrow I look forward to
- _____
- _____
- _____
- _____

Stay Positivity Journal

DATE: _____

Today I'm grateful because :

- _____
- _____
- _____

Today's Positive Affirmations / Quotes

- _____
- _____
- _____
- _____

Water Tracker

☐ 1L   ☐ 2L   ☐ 3L

Today I'm feeling   Emoji

Notes / reminders:

Something I'm proud of

- _____
- _____
- _____
- _____

Tomorrow I look forward to

- _____
- _____
- _____
- _____

Stay Positivity Journal

DATE: _____

Today I'm grateful because :
- _____
- _____
- _____

Today's Positive Affirmations / Quotes
- _____
- _____
- _____
- _____

Water Tracker
☐ 1L ☐ 2L ☐ 3L

Today I'm feeling ◯ → Emoji

Notes / reminders:

Something I'm proud of
- _____
- _____
- _____
- _____

Tomorrow I look forward to
- _____
- _____
- _____
- _____

Stay Positivity Journal

DATE: _____

Today I'm grateful because :
- _____
- _____
- _____

Today's Positive Affirmations / Quotes
- _____
- _____
- _____
- _____

Water Tracker
- ☐ 1L ☐ 2L ☐ 3L

Today I'm feeling ◯ ← **Emoji**

Notes / reminders:

Something I'm proud of
- _____
- _____
- _____
- _____

Tomorrow I look forward to
- _____
- _____
- _____
- _____

Stay Positivity Journal

DATE: _____

Today I'm grateful because :
- _____
- _____
- _____

Today's Positive Affirmations / Quotes
- _____
- _____
- _____
- _____

Water Tracker
☐ 1L   ☐ 2L   ☐ 3L

Today I'm feeling ◯ ← Emoji

Notes / reminders:

Something I'm proud of
- _____
- _____
- _____
- _____

Tomorrow I look forward to
- _____
- _____
- _____
- _____

Stay Positivity Journal

DATE: _____

Today I'm grateful because :

- _____
- _____
- _____

Today's Positive Affirmations / Quotes

- _____
- _____
- _____
- _____

Water Tracker

☐ 1L ☐ 2L ☐ 3L

Today I'm feeling ⭕ **Emoji**

Notes / reminders:

Something I'm proud of

- _____
- _____
- _____
- _____

Tomorrow I look forward to

- _____
- _____
- _____
- _____

Stay Positivity Journal

DATE: _____

Today I'm grateful because :
- _____
- _____
- _____

Today's Positive Affirmations / Quotes
- _____
- _____
- _____
- _____

Water Tracker
☐ 1L ☐ 2L ☐ 3L

Today I'm feeling ◯ ← **Emoji**

Notes / reminders:

Something I'm proud of
- _____
- _____
- _____
- _____

Tomorrow I look forward to
- _____
- _____
- _____
- _____

Stay Positivity Journal

DATE: _____

Today I'm grateful because :
- _____
- _____
- _____

Today's Positive Affirmations / Quotes
- _____
- _____
- _____
- _____

Water Tracker
☐ 1L ☐ 2L ☐ 3L

Today I'm feeling ◯ → **Emoji**

Notes / reminders:

Something I'm proud of
- _____
- _____
- _____
- _____

Tomorrow I look forward to
- _____
- _____
- _____
- _____

Stay Positivity Journal

DATE: _____

Today I'm grateful because :
- _____
- _____
- _____

Today's Positive Affirmations / Quotes
- _____
- _____
- _____
- _____

Water Tracker
☐ 1L   ☐ 2L   ☐ 3L

Today I'm feeling ◯ ← **Emoji**

Notes / reminders:

Something I'm proud of
- _____
- _____
- _____
- _____

Tomorrow I look forward to
- _____
- _____
- _____
- _____

Stay Positivity Journal

DATE: _____

Today I'm grateful because :
- _____
- _____
- _____

Today's Positive Affirmations / Quotes
- _____
- _____
- _____
- _____

Water Tracker
- ☐ 1L ☐ 2L ☐ 3L

Today I'm feeling ◯ → Emoji

Notes / reminders:

Something I'm proud of
- _____
- _____
- _____
- _____

Tomorrow I look forward to
- _____
- _____
- _____
- _____

Stay Positivity Journal

DATE: _____

Today I'm grateful because :
- _____
- _____
- _____

Today's Positive Affirmations / Quotes
- _____
- _____
- _____
- _____

Water Tracker
☐ 1L   ☐ 2L   ☐ 3L

Today I'm feeling ◯ **Emoji**

Notes / reminders:

Something I'm proud of
- _____
- _____
- _____
- _____

Tomorrow I look forward to
- _____
- _____
- _____
- _____

Made in the USA
Middletown, DE
23 December 2023